HOW TO OVERCOME DEPRESSION:

MENTAL HEALTH FOR YOUNG ADULTS

Melody N. Sommer

TABLE OF CONTENTS

INTRODUCTION

If you're reading this, you're probably a teenager or young adult looking for ways to conquer anxiety, stress and depression, or you're a parent in search of how to help your child through this tough time.

There are a lot of hormonal changes that occur in the body at puberty, and that alone could cause teens to start having unfamiliar feelings such as anxiety and depression. But it's nothing to fret about.

Whether or not those feelings are caused by hormonal changes or something else, you can overcome them. It's possible! Yes! You're going to look back at this time and be glad you didn't give up.

This book will work you through that journey of overcoming depression. They're tested and confirmed guides that helped overcome these feelings for me and some other people I know.

However, you know that you also should be ready to put in the effort. Yeah, it can be difficult sometimes but just try as much as you can, and I promise you that it'll be alright soon. Okay?

THE TRUTH ABOUT ANXIETY

It's okay, dear. You've got this. I promise you.

Everyone feels anxious sometimes, when they're faced with a difficult challenge or when things don't seem to be working as planned. For example, you may get anxious before your exams especially when you're not prepared for it, or when you're called to answer a question you don't know in class, or your first day in a new school, and so on. This feeling is normal. It's a hormonal response that prepares the body to respond quickly to these changes. Anxiety helps you prepare yourself for these changes, so there's no need to feel bad about being anxious. However, if the feeling comes so often that it starts to overwhelm you, there just might be a little problem.

I'll tell you a brief story about Sarah. She was only in seventh grade when she was diagnosed with anxiety disorder. Her parents were busy people. Her mom had a 9-5 job while her dad was an international pilot, so he was hardly around. She had her nanny, but there's nannying and there's parenting.

Sarah didn't usually do well at school. She had no friends, and would always fret about the tiniest thing. No one paid much attention to this until a new teacher in her school came. The teacher happened to also be a psychologist. She was the first to notice Sarah's disorder, and would often call her to her office to talk to her. Of course, she never spoke about the disorder to Sarah. She would only talk to her about random things to cheer her up and make her forget whatever she was anxious about at that moment. Their bond grew after several months. One day, Sarah invited the teacher over to her house. Her parents also loved the teacher, and this was when she talked to the parents about Sarah's disorder.

The parents listened. Of course, they loved their kid, so why won't they? They began to pay more attention to the little girl and discovered what usually made her anxious. When she finally opened up about what usually made her anxious, guess what she said? It wasn't even because the parents weren't there, yeah, it might have started from there but that wasn't it. She talked about things that she feared were going to happen. Things like her dad dying in a plane crash, her parents getting divorced like she'd seen happen to some of her peers, having to drop out of school because she didn't do well, and fear of getting bullied by her crush. She talked about how stressful it was to brush her teeth in the mornings, study her books, do homework, interact with friends, and do little things that didn't really matter.

You see, the thing about an anxiety disorder is that you begin to worry about everything! Things that matter, things that don't matter. Even after the 'big things' have been solved, the mins automatically shift to something else to be anxious about. Anxiety just becomes a place of solitude. That's not nice, you see. It's just not nice.

You can get better at just about everything —with effort and practice. That includes reducing anxiety.
Notice how anxiety affects your body. When you're anxious, do you feel "butterflies" in your stomach? Sweaty palms? Shaky hands? A faster heartbeat? Tight muscles?

These physical feelings are part of your body's stress response. They can be uncomfortable but they aren't harmful. You can cope. Next time you feel them, try to notice them without getting upset that they're there. You don't have to push the feelings away. But you don't have to give them all your attention either. See if you can let them be in the background.

So yeah, conquering this feeling is what I'm going to be dealing with in the next chapter.

OVERCOMING ANXIETY DISORDERS

Quick question, what've you got on your mind?

Do you have the mindset that you can't change because that's how you are? Are you comfortable about being shy so you feel there's no need to do something about it? When you feel anxious, do you just go to your space and begin to overthink or do you get up and tell yourself, "I'm not going to let this get the better of me cause I own my life"?

They say it all starts from the mind. Brain Science has proven that you can teach your brain new ways to react to the things that happen around you.

Next time you feel overwhelmed with anxiety, tell yourself that you've got this.

Believe that you're better than this and that you can overcome it.

So dear, you need to establish this mindset first before you can proceed with every other step.

Breathe, darling, just breathe.

When you feel anxious, take deep, slow breaths. You can say it out loud–breath in... breath out... in... out. Ever thought of why during exercises in school or fitness training, you're usually asked to take deep breaths? It doesn't just help with physical fitness, but also for mental fitness.

Taking slow, steady breaths slows down the release of stress hormones. It helps to ease the body and mind. It sort of deviates your attention from these anxious thoughts to the breath you're taking. As ridiculous as it might sound, it's true. It helps you feel more stable and less anxious. Slow breaths help increase your lungs, and lower your heart rate, hence allowing you to feel at rest.

You say it, then you face it!

Ever tried talking to yourself? Sure, I know you have. Everyone talks to themselves at some point. In fact, I think the most successful people on earth say a couple of things to themselves every day.

But what kind of things do you tell yourself when you feel anxious? Do you say things like, "I can't do this!" or, "What if I do this and it doesn't work out?" or, "It's just too much for me." No! You should NEVER say things like that to yourself. Instead, tell yourself I CAN and I WILL. Tell yourself that it will work, and even if it doesn't work out eventually, tell yourself that it's probably for the best. Yes, it may not have worked out as planned but it's still okay. At least, you won't live with the guilt of not trying because not trying only makes things worse.

I love writing a lot but there was a time in my life I'd refuse every opportunity I got to publish my works because I was afraid of getting regretted. There are so many opportunities I lost that I know I wouldn't have if I had just believed in myself a little more. Sure, it's not that my work would always be accepted wherever I send it, but what's worse than getting rejected is leaving with the guilt of not trying.

I know it's tough and making an effort to try could even add to the anxiety, but tell yourself that it's okay. Whether or not it eventually works out, just know that it's okay. It really is. My dear, it's all going to be fine in the end. There's always light at the end of the tunnel, only that it might take a while to reach there. But there is ALWAYS LIGHT in the end. It's all going to end well, dear. You don't have to feel anxious. You'll get through this!

Face the situation. Don't wait for anxiety to leave itself because it may not. Take it one step at a time. It won't feel difficult that way, I assure you. The more you practice, the better you get at conquering anxiety.

Let's pen down something.

One tested and trusted way to conquer anxiety is through journaling. The things you're anxious about, do you pen them down?

A friend told me the story of how journaling helped her cure anxiety. She would always pen down whatever was making her anxious no Matt how small or big. First, it always gave her that feeling of relief that happened after throwing punches at a sandbag. It was like she was transferring those problems to a paper. After she was done writing, she always felt much better. But that wasn't all. One day, she went back to read her old journals and she realized something—most of the things she wrote down as her problems had been solved. They had become things of the past. History! It was at that moment she knew that she had a lot of things to be thankful for.

Ever heard the saying, "two heads are better than one"?

You know you're not an island, right? And even an island's got water around it!

Having a social support system is important in coping with anxiety and stress. Social support groups could be useful if you're feeling lonely and don't have friends or family to rely on. Think about joining a club, a sports team, or volunteering for an organization that matters to you.

Talk to someone about it. It could be a trusted friend, your parent, a therapist–whoever. Just don't try to bottle things up. It never helps.

STRESS: A PATHWAY FOR ANXIETY

We all get stressed out sometimes, but how do you cope with stress?

One of the major reasons for anxiety is stress. Teenagers are growing adults, hence are prone to stress like an adult. Most teens experience the kind of stress that leads to anxiety when they feel a situation is dangerous, difficult, or harmful. It happens when they feel they do not have the resources to cope with these situations.

Examples of situations like this are school demands and frustration from classmates, certain changes in their bodies especially during puberty, negative thoughts, unsafe environments, family problems, involvement in too many activities at a time, high expectations, and so on.

Too high expectations and changes (both hormonal and environmental changes) are the most common causes of stress among teenagers.

Here's the story of Clara who had to change school because she wasn't doing well in the previous school. The parents felt it was because the school didn't have enough resources to take care of the students, so they enrolled her in a more reputable school where they had to pay a lot of money for school fees. They expected a lot from her. Better academic performance, making new and better friends, and all that stuff. Unfortunately, she didn't meet up to these expectations. Rather, her performance declined even more especially since there was greater competition, and it was difficult making new friends and adapting to the new environment. Everything just became so stressful and overwhelming for her.

OVERCOMING STRESS

Hey! Stir up the mind with some exercise!

Constantly moving your body can help if you're feeling stressed. A study made among students in the university discovered that engaging in aerobic exercise 2 days a week significantly lowered the overall stress including stress due to uncertainty. Several other studies have proved that participating in physical activities and exercises reduces stress levels and improves mood whereas sedentary behavior may cause increased stress, bad mood, and restlessness.

Gentle activities such as walking, jogging, biking, aerobics, and yoga go a long way in reducing stress. It should be an activity you love and enjoy doing so that you won't have to feel like another chore or stress to you.

How often do you get to rest, dear?

Teenagers need sleep to maintain good physical, mental and social health including reducing stress. It helps them to concentrate more and quickens their memory. Lack of sleep can make it harder for you to get along well with your peers, control your emotions, pay attention and perform well in class.

A good teenage sleep pattern would be:

- An average of 8-10 hours of sleep each night.
- On school days and weekends, try to wake up no more than two hours apart. This maintains the body clock's regularity.
- When you awaken in the morning, get up instead of staying in bed.
- Avoid using screens an hour before going to bed and instead engage in unwinding activities like reading, listening to music, or taking a warm

shower. Put electronic devices far away from you when about to sleep. You could leave it in another room.

- Limit daytime naps to 20 minutes or less, and take them in the early afternoon.
- Make sure you have a good atmosphere for sleep. I suggest a peaceful, low light environment.

What's your diet like?

According to studies, persons who consume a diet heavy in ultra-processed foods and added sugar are more likely to perceive their stress levels as being higher. Your diet affects every aspect of your health, including helping to reduce stress.

Chronic stress may cause you to overeat and gravitate toward sweet food and junk, which could be detrimental to your general health and mood. A lack of nutrients like magnesium and B vitamins, which are necessary for controlling stress and mood, may raise your risk of deficiency in these nutrients. Your body can be better nourished if you consume fewer highly processed meals and beverages and more whole foods like vegetables, fruits, legumes, seafood, nuts, and seeds. Thus, you might become more stress-resistant as a result.

Let's talk about your habits.

What are your habits like? What do you do when you feel extremely stressed out? How do you start your day? Do you take excess caffeine to help you concentrate when studying or do you hide in a corner to sniff some stuff you shouldn't when you feel stressed?

Watch out for those bad habits and try to replace them with good ones. I know it's not easy, and it's okay. But you know you need to put in some effort, right? You don't want the stress to get out of hand, do you?

Here are some habits to learn and unlearn:

- Start your day off right by going for a stroll in the morning and eating a nutritious breakfast.
- Avoid caffeine in the late afternoon and evening, especially in coffee, tea, chocolate, and cola.
- Steer clear of alcohol, tobacco, and illegal drugs. The truth is, these things don't help. Yeah, you might feel better for a while but trust me, it's causing a lot of damage. You wouldn't want to go to rehab or jail, would you?
- Learn relaxation exercises. Simple exercises like taking long steady breaths, going for a stroll, swimming, and so on can go a long way
- Learn to express your feelings in a polite, assertive, and clear way. If someone does something you don't like, say it. You don't have to be rude or violent with your words. You could

use phrases like "I don't like it when you yell at me, so would you lower your voice, please?"

- Practice how to handle stressful sceneries even before they come. One example is signing up for speech lessons if you experience anxiety when speaking in front of a crowd. Reduce negative self-talk by challenging bad thoughts with neutral, constructive, or alternate thinking. "My life will never get better" can be changed to "I may feel hopeless right now, but if I work at it and obtain some support, my life will get better."
- Instead of expecting perfection from yourself and others, learn to feel good about accomplishing a competent or "good enough" job.
- Take a break from stressful situations. Stress-relieving activities include things like listening to music, chatting with a friend, writing, drawing, and playing with a pet.

- Build a network of friends who help you cope positively.

Practice self-care. Truth is, it's still the little things that matter most.

Studies show that people who engage in self-care report lower levels of stress and improved quality of life, while a lack of self-care is associated with a higher risk of stress and burnout (35Trusted Source, 36Trusted Source, 37Trusted Source).

Self-care doesn't have to be elaborate or complicated. It simply means doing things that stir up happiness, and hence reducing stress. It could be as simple as an outdoor exercise, taking a bath, inhaling candle scent (aromatherapy), reading a good book, stretching before bed, getting a massage, engaging in a hobby, utilizing a diffuser with calming scents, and doing yoga. Some recommended candle scents include rose, lavender, neroli, frankincense, geranium, sandalwood, orange and Roman chamomile.

Boundaries: Humans are like elastic; we all have a breaking point.

Set boundaries and practice saying no. Some pressures are out of your control, but not all of them. Overcommitting yourself could result in a higher stress level and less time available for self-care. Being in charge of your personal life can help you feel less stressed and safeguard your mental health.

Saying "no" more frequently might be one method to do this. This is particularly important to remember if you frequently take on more than you can manage because juggling multiple obligations might make you feel overburdened. If you feel showing up for that friend's party or teen's hangout will add to your workload rather than making you relaxed, decline politely. It's okay not to always show up. It doesn't make you a bad friend. It simply makes you human, you see. If they are indeed your friend, they would understand. You're growing adults, and trust me, there'll be times when you become full adults that saying no will become a necessity. It's a habit you'd need. It might seem difficult at the beginning, but with time, it will get a lot easier.

Stress levels can be decreased by being cautious about what you take on and saying "no" to things that would unnecessarily add to your workload. By refusing to accept more than you can handle, you can establish healthy limits in your life. One strategy to manage your stress is to say "no."

Procrastination is a no-no!

Keeping track of your priorities and avoiding procrastination are two other ways to manage your stress. Your productivity could suffer if you procrastinate, leaving you with little time to make up for lost time. Stress might result from this, which is bad for your health and the quality of your sleep.

Developing the practice of creating a to-do list that is prioritized may be helpful if you frequently procrastinate. Take it bit by bit. We call it baby steps. And try not to stuff your to-do list with a lot of things you know you can't finish within the given period. Set a reasonable deadline for the number of things and proceed to the list. It's also recommended that you write your to-do list the previous night so that when you wake the next morning, you don't feel confused or overwhelmed with what to do next.

Give yourself undisturbed time to work on the tasks that must be completed today. Multitasking or switching between things can be stressful in and of itself.

DEPRESSION

First of all, depression isn't a sign of weakness. I'd like you to know that.

A couple of years ago, I graduated from high school. I couldn't attend college for one reason or another. It wasn't that I didn't want to attend college. Damn! I was smart and intelligent but I just couldn't due to personal reasons. I would watch my mates go to school and look at their college pictures on social media. This made me often sad, and gradually I became depressed. Some nights, I would wake up crying. Sometimes, I wouldn't feel like doing anything. I'd feel too tired to get out of bed, freshen up, eat, and walk from the bedroom to the living room. Sometimes, I could even get too tired to change my lying posture in bed. It was that bad. I would often think of suicide but I tried hard not to give it a second thought because I'm a Christian and it's totally against my faith.

My faith helped me a lot to overcome depression, but since this isn't a spiritual book, I'll be giving other ways that also helped me.

PS: I'll save the spiritual method I used to conquer depression for another book. You can stay updated on that.

Depression can be really bad which is why the moment you notice any symptom of depression, it's important you fight it. One very effective way to do so is by opening up to a loved one. I'll buttress more on that in the next chapter.

Here, I'll be talking about the most common symptoms of depression.

- Persistent mood swings and sadness: Depression is often characterized by persistent crying and having an overwhelming feeling of hopelessness. Teenagers with depression, however, might not always seem depressed. Instead, tension, wrath, and irritation may be the most noticeable signs.

- Difficulties at school: Low energy and trouble concentrating are two symptoms of depression. This could affect a student's performance at school by causing low attendance, a reduction in grades, or irritation with their homework.

- Lack of motivation: You don't have the motivation or energy to do anything. The things you used to love no longer matter to you. You lack the zeal to do anything. You probably just want to stay in bed all day with a duvet wrapped over you. You just want to isolate yourself from everyone. Staying in your space is very important, true, but when it becomes too often that even in your space you still lack energy, it could be a sign of depression.

- Drug and alcohol abuse: Teenagers who are depressed may try to self-medicate by using alcohol or drugs. Unfortunately, drug misuse only worsens the situation.
- Low self-esteem: Study has shown that extreme feelings of shyness, feeling of shame, unworthiness and failure are all signs of depression. You choose not to participate in an activity because you feel you'd suck at it. You don't feel worthy of other people's love, respect or care, hence, you hide in your shadow. That's not true, dear. You're worthy of all the love the world has to offer.
- Screen and phone addiction: Surprised? Nah, I don't expect you to be. Teens could stick to their phones or watch tv all day in an attempt to escape your troubles, but frequent smartphone and Internet use would only make you feel more alone and lonely.

- Recklessness: Teenagers who are depressed may engage in risky or harmful behaviors including drunk driving, binge drinking, unsafe sex or may be violent with others. Teens who have been victims of bullying may become hostile and violent themselves in an attempt to hide the part of them that has gone sour due to bullying.

- Unexpected changes in nutrition and sleep: You may sleep more than normal or, conversely, struggle with insomnia. You feel restless whenever it's bedtime. Also, you often stress-eat. You take a lot of junk or sometimes, you lose your appetite entirely. Sometimes, you either lose too much weight or gain excess weight.

- Suicidal thoughts: You begin to contemplate suicide. You feel there's nothing left to live for. You tell yourself things like,"why don't I just die and end this?" You just want to give up because you see no value left in your life. But that should never be it because it's a lie.

There are several other symptoms including overreacting, social awkwardness, anxiety, poor hygiene, memory loss etc. However, it doesn't mean that if you show one or two of these symptoms, you're automatically proven to be depressed. No. Other things are also considered. But it's always important to take care of your mental health.

OVERCOMING DEPRESSION

What's your early morning routine?

Simple steps like praying, making your bed, positive self-talk, and helping out with morning chores go a long way in starting your day refreshing. Other morning routines that we often take for granted but are necessary include:

JOURNALING
When you wake up, writing down your thoughts, your blessings, your daily goals, and your affirmations will help you rediscover your sense of self.

SUNLIGHT:
Do you get up during summer mornings to watch the moon pave way for the sun? Do you step out to get a dose of a nice early morning sun?

Get as much natural light as possible during the day, especially in the morning. This will help the body produce melatonin at the right times in the sleep cycle. Exposing yourself to bright sunlight for 30 minutes a day helps keep your internal clock set. The exposure must come through the eyes though! This helps the circadian rhythm, which is what regulates the sleep and wake cycles and ensures a good night's sleep. This helps both physical and mental health.

AEROBIC EXERCISE

A 10-minute walk can improve your mood for two hours. The key to sustaining these mood benefits is to exercise regularly. Activities should be moderately intense- you do not need to sweat strenuously to see results. It is important that when finding exercises they are continuous and rhythmic. Walking, swimming, dancing, biking, and running are all great examples.

MEDITATION

Taking about 10-20 minutes to meditate every morning goes a long way in conquering depression. You might want to sit and close your eyes to focus better. Takc deep slow breaths and give yourself room to feel your thoughts. Don't push the thoughts away. Allow yourself to feel it. Stay with it until you find yourself controlling it. It is advisable to have a mantra when meditating to help you focus your thoughts more by yourself. You might not get it the first few times, but after a while, you'll get better at it. You can also see a meditation expert teach you how to meditate.

HEALTHY EATING

The food you consume directly affects how you feel, especially breakfast. Your teen's mood can be improved by cutting back on items like caffeine, sugar, alcohol, trans fats, and highly processed foods that can have a detrimental impact on your brain and emotions.

Have fun! Socialize. Remember you only live life once.

As a teenager or young adult, it's important to socialize and have fun. Humans are social beings after all. You don't have to engage in heavy discussions if you don't want to, but simple things like playing games, chitchats, organizing a picnic etc help you lighten up the mood. Isolation can be reduced even by simply spending time with others. Face-to-face communication should be used for this, not online. Also, this should be done as often as possible.

Cuddling and touch are really underrated ways of easing the mood. I remember one night. It was my birthday night but nothing went as planned that day. The day started with my phone screen damaging. Just like that. The screen just stopped working. As if that wasn't enough, there were a lot of canceled plans during the day. Then, in the evening I was trying to talk to a friend over the phone but the call only ended in more tears. I went to my sister's room. She was already asleep because it was about 1 am already. I turned my head the other way to get some sleep but I remained there for about half an hour. I wasn't sleepy. I was totally restless and sad. So, I turned to face her and just held her close. I felt the entire weight drop, and in less than ten minutes, I'd fallen asleep. Just like that. It felt like magic. It was like I'd given her a portion of my sorrows. Of course, she had no idea because she was asleep.

The best place to be is with nature!

Spend some time with nature and animals. Studies show that being in nature and spending time in green spaces like parks and forests are beneficial strategics to conquer depression. You can go family camping on weekends, look for green areas like neighborhood parks and your school garden and stay for about an hour or two. You may do your homework there or study.

Having a pet also helps to improve your mood. Your body releases oxytocin, a hormone that helps to boost the mood when you touch or snuggle a pet. Dogs, especially, have a way of lightening up the mood because they have some human character in them. It also helps to reduce loneliness and feel companionship. Imagine having a dog that comes to hug you when you return from school. Or a cute harmless cat that snuggles with you in bed. Or a parrot that repeats every word you say.

Little things that matter.

Sometimes, it's the little things you do that lighten up your mood. Things like laughing at silly jokes, and engaging in hobbies such as painting, writing, reading, dancing, singing, sports, cooking, and so on, go a long way in overcoming depression. Ever felt the sense of satisfaction that comes with showing a little act of kindness? Maybe assisting an elderly person in crossing the road or assisting someone with their bags or sharing your food/snacks with a hungry person. Little things like that matter a lot, not just for the person you're helping out but also for yourself.

Coping with suicidal thoughts.

Seek assistance the moment you feel the depressive feeling become so severe that you see no other option except to hurt yourself or others. It might be quite challenging to reach out to someone you trust when you're experiencing such intense feelings, but it's important that you do so—it could be a friend, a member of your family, or a teacher. Call a suicide helpline if you don't feel like you have somebody to talk to or if you think it might be easier to talk to a stranger. You'll be able to communicate openly with someone who comprehends your situation and can support you in overcoming your emotions.

Whatever the circumstance, facing death and pulling back from the edge require tremendous guts. You can draw strength from that bravery to push forward and get over your depression.

Even if you can't see it now, there is ALWAYS another option. Many survivors of suicide attempts claim that they attempted suicide because they erroneously believed there was no other way to solve an issue they were having. Even though they couldn't see a way out at the time, they didn't want to die. No matter how horrible you feel, just keep in mind that these feelings will pass. It does not make you a bad or weak person if you have thoughts of harming yourself or other people. You may experience thoughts and feelings that are abnormal due to depression. If you are brave enough to express your feelings, no one would blame or judge you for them.

Tell yourself to wait for a day before acting if your emotions are out of control. This can allow you some time to reflect carefully and detach yourself from the intense feelings that are bothering you. Try to chat to someone, anyone, as long as they are not another sad or suicidal individual. Speak to your parents or a trusted person or dial a hotline. Yeah, it could seem difficult but it's not impossible. Just try to do it. Never forget that there's always someone who cares, always.

Positive energy! Positive vibes only!

Yes, remind yourself about these things often. Think about that time when they all said you couldn't do it, but you did it anyway. Remember that time they clapped for you in class for answering the question correctly. Recall that smile your momma and papa gave you when you did something right. Have you forgotten that hobby and how you're so good at it? These are gentle reminders that should always come in handy for you.

Goodness! You're a badass. You're lovely. You know the things you do and do well. So what if someone does better than you in class? Have you already forgotten the stuff you are good at? I bet the person doesn't come near. You see, you're special. You're lovely. You've accomplished a lot of things you overlook. How about you take a moment and think back on those things? The moment you start to notice what's good is the moment you start to feel good.

Again, seek help. No one's an island, and even islands have water around them.

Opening up about how you're feeling might be challenging, particularly if you're experiencing feelings of worthlessness, humiliation, or depression. It's crucial to keep in mind that many people experience feelings similar to these from time to time; this does not imply that you are weak, inherently flawed, or unworthy of praise. You'll feel less alone if you accept your emotions and talk to a trusted person about them.

People do love and care about you, although it may not feel that way right now. If you have the bravery to discuss your depression with someone, it can and will get better. Some individuals believe that talking about difficult emotions would make them worse, yet this is virtually never the case. Sharing your troubles with someone who will listen and care about what you have to say is very beneficial. They only need to be good listeners; they don't need to be able to "fix" you.

Find a different adult you can trust if your parents are being abusive in any manner or have their own problems you wouldn't want to add to. Other adults you can approach are a relative, teachers, counselors, or coaches. This person can either direct you to the support you require or assist you in approaching your parents. Also, several hotlines, programs, and support groups are available if you really have no one you can talk to. Talk to someone no matter what, especially if you are considering hurting yourself or others. The most courageous thing you can do is to ask for assistance. It is also the first step toward recovery.

<u>NOTE</u>: There are several other ways to conquer depression that were not dealt with in this chapter, such as healthy dieting, exercise, breathing etc, but were dealt with in the previous chapters. They all help to boost mood and conquer depression.

CONCLUSION

Adolescence is a critical time for forming social and emotional habits that are necessary for mental health. Develop coping, problem-solving, and interpersonal skills as well as appropriate sleep and exercise routines. Learn to control your emotions. It is crucial to create safe and encouraging conditions in the home, at school, and in the larger community.

Parents should seek medical help for their teenagers suffering from depression if the situation gets worse.

Most importantly, as teens and young adults, you've got to be compassionate and nice to yourself if you're experiencing anxiety, stress and/or depression. Know you're not alone in your struggles. Don't be too hard on yourself.

Healing takes time!